Table of Contents

Introduction 3
    MIND Diet 3
    Foods To Eat On The MIND Diet 4
    Foods To Avoid On The MIND Diet 6
    A Sample Meal Plan For One Week 8
Research On The MIND Diet And Brain Health 13
Recipes 14
    Blueberry-Walnut Pancakes 14
    Creamy Zucchini Noodles With White Lentil Spring Onion Sauce 16
    CHEESY SUNFLOWER SPRINKLE INGREDIENTS 17
    Ikarian Longevity Stew With Black Eyed Peas 19
    Greek Chicken Thighs With Artichokes And Olives 20
    Pecan-Crusted Chicken 23
    Crunchy Walnut-Crusted Salmon Fillets 24
    Mussels Three Ways 26
    Roasted Ginger Salmon 29
    Spinach And Cranberry Stuffed Salmon 32
    Triple-Citrus Ginger Black Cod 33
    Arugula, Strawberry And Walnut Salad 36
    Barley Stuffed Tomato With Caramelized Vegetables .. 38
    Brandon's Roasted Broccoli 40

Latin Style Kale 42

Sweet And Sour Sesame Asian Cabbage And Kale 44

Indian Greens 46

Mediterranean Greens 48

Golden Roasted Cauliflower 50

Ikarian Tabouli Salad 51

Introduction

The MIND diet is designed to prevent dementia and loss of brain function as you age. It combines the Mediterranean diet and the DASH diet to create a dietary pattern that focuses specifically on brain health. This book is a detailed guide for beginners, with everything you need to know about the MIND diet and how to follow it.

MIND Diet

MIND stands for the Mediterranean-DASH Intervention for Neurodegenerative Delay. The MIND diet aims to reduce dementia and the decline in brain health that often occurs as people get older. It combines aspects of two very popular diets, the Mediterranean diet and the Dietary Approaches to Stop Hypertension (DASH) diet. Many experts regard the Mediterranean and DASH diets as some of the healthiest. Research has shown they can lower blood pressure and reduce the risk of heart disease, diabetes and several other diseases. But researchers wanted to create a diet specifically to help improve brain function and prevent dementia. To do this, they combined foods from the Mediterranean and DASH diets that had been shown to benefit brain health. For example, both the Mediterranean and DASH diets recommend eating a lot of fruit. Fruit intake has not been correlated with improved brain function, but eating berries has been. Thus, the MIND diet encourages its followers to eat berries, but does not emphasize consuming fruit in general. Currently, there are no set guidelines for how to follow the MIND diet. Simply eat more of the 10 foods the diet encourages you to eat, and eat less of the five foods the diet recommends you limit.

Foods To Eat On The MIND Diet

Here are the foods the MIND diet encourages:

• Green, leafy vegetables: Aim for six or more servings per week. This includes kale, spinach, cooked greens and salads.

• All other vegetables: Try to eat another vegetable in addition to the green leafy vegetables at least once a day. It is best to choose non-starchy vegetables because they have a lot of nutrients with a low number of calories.

• Berries: Eat berries at least twice a week. Although the published research only includes strawberries, you should also consume other berries like blueberries, raspberries and blackberries for their antioxidant benefits.

• Nuts: Try to get five servings of nuts or more each week. The creators of the MIND diet don't specify what kind of nuts to consume, but it is probably best to vary the type of nuts you eat to obtain a variety of nutrients.

• Olive oil: Use olive oil as your main cooking oil.

• Whole grains: Aim for at least three servings daily. Choose whole grains like oatmeal, quinoa, brown rice, whole-wheat pasta and 100% whole-wheat bread.

• Fish: Eat fish at least once a week. It is best to choose fatty fish like salmon, sardines, trout, tuna and mackerel for their high amounts of omega-3 fatty acids.

• Beans: Include beans in at least four meals every week. This includes all beans, lentils and soybeans.

• Poultry: Try to eat chicken or turkey at least twice a week. Note that fried chicken is not encouraged on the MIND diet.

• Wine: Aim for no more than one glass daily. Both red and white wine may benefit the brain. However, much research has focused on the red wine compound resveratrol, which may help protect against Alzheimer's disease.

If you are unable to consume the targeted amount of servings, don't quit the MIND diet altogether. Research has shown that following the MIND diet even a moderate amount is associated with a reduced risk of Alzheimer's disease. When you're following the diet, you can eat more than just these 10 foods. However, the more you stick to the diet, the better your results may be. According to research, eating more of the 10 recommended foods and less of the foods to avoid has been associated with a lower risk of Alzheimer's disease, and better brain function over time.

Foods To Avoid On The MIND Diet

The MIND diet recommends limiting the following five foods:

• Butter and margarine: Try to eat less than 1 tablespoon (about 14 grams) daily. Instead, try using olive oil as your primary cooking fat, and dipping your bread in olive oil with herbs.

• Cheese: The MIND diet recommends limiting your cheese consumption to less than once per week.

• Red meat: Aim for no more than three servings each week. This includes all beef, pork, lamb and products made from these meats.

• Fried food: The MIND diet highly discourages fried food, especially the kind from fast-food restaurants. Limit your consumption to less than once per week.

• Pastries and sweets: This include most of the processed junk food and desserts you can think of. Ice cream, cookies, brownies, snack cakes, donuts, candy and more. Try to limit these to no more than four times a week.

Researchers encourage limiting your consumption of these foods because they contain saturated fats and trans fats. Studies have found that trans fats are clearly associated with all sorts of diseases, including heart disease and even Alzheimer's disease. However, the health effects of saturated fat are widely debated in the nutrition world. Although the research on saturated fats and heart disease may be inconclusive and highly contested, animal research and observational studies in humans do suggest that consuming saturated fats in excess is associated with poor brain health.

A Sample Meal Plan For One Week

Making meals for the MIND diet doesn't have to be complicated. Here's a seven-day meal plan to get you started:

Monday

- Breakfast: Greek yogurt with raspberries, topped with sliced almonds.

- Lunch: Mediterranean salad with olive-oil-based dressing, grilled chicken, whole-wheat pita.

- Dinner: Burrito bowl with brown rice, black beans, fajita vegetables, grilled chicken, salsa and guacamole.

Tuesday

- Breakfast: Wheat toast with almond butter, scrambled eggs.

- Lunch: Grilled chicken sandwich, blackberries, carrots.

- Dinner: Grilled salmon, side salad with olive-oil-based dressing, brown rice.

Wednesday

- Breakfast: Steel-cut oatmeal with strawberries, hard-boiled eggs.

- Lunch: Mexican-style salad with mixed greens, black beans, red onion, corn, grilled chicken and olive-oil-based dressing.

- Dinner: Chicken and vegetable stir-fry, brown rice.

Thursday

- Breakfast: Greek yogurt with peanut butter and banana.

- Lunch: Baked trout, collard greens, black-eyed peas.

- Dinner: Whole-wheat spaghetti with turkey meatballs and marinara sauce, side salad with olive-oil-based dressing.

Friday

- Breakfast: Wheat toast with avocado, omelet with peppers and onions.

- Lunch: Chili made with ground turkey.

- Dinner: Greek-seasoned baked chicken, oven-roasted potatoes, side salad, wheat dinner roll.

Saturday

- Breakfast: Overnight oats with strawberries.

- Lunch: Fish tacos on whole wheat tortillas, brown rice, pinto beans.

- Dinner: Chicken gyro on whole-wheat pita, cucumber and tomato salad.

Sunday

- Breakfast: Spinach frittata, sliced apple and peanut butter.

- Lunch: Tuna salad sandwich on wheat bread, plus carrots and celery with hummus.

- Dinner: Curry chicken, brown rice, lentils.

You can drink a glass of wine with each dinner to satisfy the MIND diet recommendations. Nuts can also make a great snack. Most salad dressings you find at the store are not made primarily with olive oil, but you can easily make your own salad dressing at home. To make a simple balsamic vinaigrette, combine three parts extra virgin olive oil with one-part balsamic vinegar. Add a little Dijon mustard, salt and pepper, then mix well.

The MIND Diet May Decrease Oxidative Stress And Inflammation

The current research on the MIND diet has not been able to show exactly how it works. However, the scientists who created the diet think it may work by reducing oxidative stress and inflammation. Oxidative stress occurs when unstable molecules called free radicals accumulate in the body in large quantities. This often causes damage to cells. The brain is especially vulnerable to this type of damage. Inflammation is your body's natural response to injury and infection. But if it's not properly regulated, inflammation can also be harmful and contribute to many chronic diseases. Together, oxidative stress and inflammation can be quite detrimental to the brain. In recent years, they've been the focus of some interventions to prevent and treat Alzheimer's disease. Following the Mediterranean and DASH diets has been associated with lower levels of oxidative stress and inflammation. Because the MIND diet is a hybrid of these two diets, the foods that make up the MIND diet probably also have antioxidant and anti-inflammatory effects. The antioxidants in berries and the vitamin E in olive oil, green leafy vegetables and nuts are thought to benefit brain function by protecting the brain from oxidative stress. Additionally, the omega-3 fatty acids found in fatty fish are well-known for their ability to lower inflammation in the brain, and have been associated with slower loss of brain function.

The Mind Diet May Reduce Harmful Beta-Amyloid Proteins

Researchers also believe the MIND diet may benefit the brain by reducing potentially harmful beta-amyloid proteins. Beta-amyloid proteins are protein fragments found naturally in the body. However, they can accumulate and form plaques that build up in the brain, disrupting communication between brain cells and eventually leading to brain cell death. In fact, many scientists believe these plaques are one of the primary causes of Alzheimer's disease. Animal and test-tube studies suggest that the antioxidants and vitamins that many MIND diet foods contain may help prevent the formation of beta-amyloid plaques in the brain. Additionally, the MIND diet limits foods that contain saturated fats and trans fats, which studies have shown can increase beta-amyloid protein levels in mice's brains. Human observational studies have found that consuming these fats was associated with a doubled risk of Alzheimer's disease. However, it is important to note that this type of research is not able to determine cause and effect. Higher-quality, controlled studies are needed to discover exactly how the MIND diet may benefit brain health.

Research On The MIND Diet And Brain Health

The MIND diet hasn't been around very long — the first official paper on the diet was published in 2015. So, it's no surprise there's not much research investigating its effects. However, two observational studies on the MIND diet have shown very promising results. In one study of 923 older adults, people who followed the MIND diet the closest had a 53% lower risk of Alzheimer's disease than people who followed it the least. Interestingly, people who followed the MIND diet only moderately still seemed to benefit from it, and cut their risk of Alzheimer's disease by 35%, on average. The second study found that people who followed the MIND diet the closest experienced a slower decline in brain function compared to people who followed the diet the least. However, note that both these studies were observational, meaning they can't prove cause and effect. They can only detect associations. So, while the early research is promising, it can't say for sure that the MIND diet caused the reduced risk of Alzheimer's disease or the slower brain decline. However, researchers recently received approval to start a controlled study on the effects of the MIND diet. While this study won't be completed for several years, this is a big step toward determining if the MIND diet directly benefits brain function.

Recipes

Blueberry-Walnut Pancakes

Ingredients

- 3 large omega-3 eggs

- 3/4 cup almond milk

- 1/2 tablespoon freshly squeezed lemon juice

- 1 teaspoon vanilla extract

- ½ cup coconut flour

- 1/2 teaspoon baking powder

- 1/2 teaspoon baking soda

- pinch of sea salt

- 1/4 cup roughly chopped walnuts

- coconut oil, for greasing the skillet (about 1/4 cup)

- 1/2 cup arrowroot powder

- 1 teaspoon of cinnamon

- 1-pint fresh blueberries

Preparation

- In a large bowl, whisk the eggs and then add the almond milk, lemon juice, and vanilla. Whisk until well blended.

- In a separate bowl, mix together the coconut flour, cinnamon, baking powder, baking soda, salt, and arrowroot. Add the dry ingredients to the wet mixture, 1/4 cup at a time, while continuously whisking. Once combined, gently fold in the walnuts.

- Grease a large skillet and place over medium heat. Once the skillet is hot, use a ladle to pour 3-inch pancakes onto the skillet. Cook until bubbles appear, then flip. The pancake should cook on each side for about 2-3 minutes.

Repeat with rest of the batter. Add a tablespoon or more of coconut oil to the hot griddle, as needed.

• Make a blueberry sauce by simmering the blueberries in a small saucepan with 2 tablespoons of water for 10 minutes before serving.

• To serve, place 3 pancakes on a plate and top each stack with the blueberry sauce.

Creamy Zucchini Noodles With White Lentil Spring Onion Sauce

Ingredients

• 1/3 cup white lentils, picked over + rinsed

• 3/4 cup roughly chopped spring onion greens (like chives, green onions or ramp greens; or a mix)

• 1/4 cup basil leaves

• 2 tablespoons olive oil

• 2 tablespoons filtered water

• 1 teaspoon lemon zest

• 1 tablespoon fresh lemon juice

• 1 teaspoon mellow/light miso

- 1/4 teaspoon pure maple syrup/agave nectar

- sea salt and ground black pepper, to taste

NOODLE INGREDIENTS

- 4 medium zucchinis

- roasted vegetables

- extra basil, chopped, for garnish

CHEESY SUNFLOWER SPRINKLE INGREDIENTS

- 1/3 cup raw, unsalted sunflower seeds

- 1 teaspoon nutritional yeast

- 1/2 teaspoon sea salt

- 1/4 teaspoon garlic powder

- 1/4 teaspoon mellow/light miso

Directions

- Start by bringing a medium saucepan of water to a boil over medium-high heat. Add the lentils to the water and stir. Bring the lentils back up to a hearty simmer. Cook the lentils until slightly mushy, about 25 minutes. Drain the lentils and transfer them to the bowl of a food processor.

• To the food processor bowl, add the chopped spring onion greens, basil, olive oil, water, lemon zest, lemon juice, miso, maple syrup, salt, and pepper. Run the motor of the food processor on high until you have a smooth and creamy consistency, stopping to scrape the sides down a couple times. Check the sauce for seasoning, adjust, and set aside.

• Run the zucchinis through a spiralizer or make strands out of them with a julienne peeler. Place zucchini noodles in a large bowl. Toss zucchini noodles with the spring onion miso sauce, and some salt and pepper to taste. Once noodles are coated, divide them among 4 serving bowls. Top the creamy zucchini noodles with the cheesy sunflower sprinkle, roasted vegetables, and chopped basil. Serve immediately.

CHEESY SUNFLOWER SPRINKLE DIRECTIONS

• Combine the sunflower seeds, nutritional yeast, salt, garlic powder, and miso in the bowl of a food processor.

• Run the motor of the food processor on high until you have a crumbly, dusty consistency.

• Transfer cheesy sunflower sprinkle to another bowl, wipe the food processor bowl out with a dry towel, and return it to the base.

Ikarian Longevity Stew With Black Eyed Peas
Ingredients

• ½ cup extra virgin olive oil

• 1 large red onion, finely chopped

• 4 garlic cloves, finely chopped

• 1 fennel bulb

• 1 cup (8 ounces) black eyed peas (with dried peas, bring to a boil, boil for 1 minute, remove from heat, cover and let sit for an hour. Drain, rinse, and use.)

• 1 large, firm ripe tomato, finely chopped

• 2 tsp tomato paste, diluted in ¼ cup water

• 2 bay leaves

• salt to taste

• 1 bunch dill, finely chopped

Directions

• Heat half the olive oil over medium heat and cook the onion, garlic, and fennel bulb stirring occasionally, until soft (about 12 minutes). Add the black-eyed peas and toss to coat in the oil.

• Add the tomato, tomato paste and enough water to cover the beans by about an inch. Add the bay leaves. Bring to a boil, reduce heat and simmer until the black-eyed peas are about half way cooked. (Check after 40 minutes, but it may take over an hour.)

• Add the chopped dill and season with salt.

• Continue cooking until the black-eyed peas are tender. Remove, pour in remaining raw olive oil and serve.

Greek Chicken Thighs With Artichokes And Olives
Ingredients

• 8 bone-in, skin-on chicken thighs (about 2 1/2 pounds)

• 1/4 teaspoon sea salt

• 1/4 teaspoon freshly ground black pepper

• 1/4 teaspoon granulated garlic

• 1 medium onion

- 2 1/2 tablespoons extra-virgin olive oil, divided

- 3 large garlic cloves, finely chopped

- 1 can (15 ounces) water-packed artichoke hearts, drained

- 4 ounces mixed, pitted Greek olives

- 1 1/2 cup low-sodium chicken broth

- 2 tablespoons fresh chopped oregano leaves (or 2 teaspoons dried oregano)

- 1 large lemon, sliced into thin rounds (preferably Meyer lemon)

- 2 tablespoons water

- 1 tablespoon arrowroot starch

Preparation

- Trim any excess fat from the chicken thighs. Season the chicken with the salt, pepper, and granulated garlic.

- Cut the onion in half through the root end. Peel, then lay the onion flat on a cutting board and slice crosswise into thin half-moons.

• Heat 1 1/2 tablespoons of the oil in a heavy, wide-mouthed pan (3- to 4-quart braiser or sauté pan with a lid) over medium heat. When the oil is hot, add the chicken, skin side down. Cook until the skin is crisp and golden brown, 7 to 9 minutes. Remove the chicken thighs from the pan to a plate or rimmed baking sheet and set aside.

• To the same pan, add the onions and cook until softened, 3 to 4 minutes. Then add the chopped garlic and cook 1 minute more. Add the artichoke hearts, olives, broth, remaining olive oil, and oregano. Add the chicken thighs back into the pan and top the chicken with the lemon slices.

• Bring the mixture to a strong simmer, put the lid on, and reduce the heat to medium-low. Simmer over low heat for 12 to 13 minutes or until the thighs reach an internal temperature of 165°F when measured with a digital thermometer.

• To serve, place the chicken thighs in shallow bowls and pour the vegetables and jus over the top. If you prefer thicker gravy, whisk together 1 tablespoon arrowroot starch and 1 tablespoon cold water in a small bowl until smooth. Remove the chicken thighs from the pan and stir the arrowroot mixture into the juices and stir. Cook for 1 to 2 minutes, until the juices thicken into gravy.

Pecan-Crusted Chicken

Ingredients

- 4 boneless skinless chicken breasts, 6 to 8 oz. each

- 1 1/2 teaspoons salt, divided

- 1 teaspoon lemon juice

- 1 1/2 cups plain yogurt

- 2 tablespoons Dijon mustard

- 2 cups pecans, finely chopped

- 1 cup bread crumbs

- olive oil for sautéing

Preparation

- Use a mallet to pound chicken breasts into a uniform 1/2-inch thickness. Cut each breast into 2 or 3 pieces for manageability.

- Combine lemon juice, yogurt, mustard, and 1/2 teaspoon salt in a bowl and set aside. Put chicken pieces in mixture and let sit for about 10 minutes.

- Combine pecans, crumbs, and 1 teaspoon salt in a bowl and set aside.

- Heat about 1 tablespoon olive oil in a sauté pan over medium high heat. Wipe excess yogurt off chicken and dredge in pecan mixture. When oil is hot, add chicken pieces to pan and cook about 3-4 minutes on each side until golden brown on the outside and cooked through. You may need to do it in batches, in which case you should wipe the pan out between batches and add a bit more oil.

- Serve immediately.

Crunchy Walnut-Crusted Salmon Fillets
Ingredients

- 1 1/2 cups California walnuts

- 3 tablespoons dry breadcrumbs

- 3 tablespoons lemon rind, finely grated

- 1 1/2 tablespoons extra-virgin olive oil

- 3 tablespoons fresh dill, chopped

- Salt and pepper to taste

- 6 3-ounce salmon fillets, skin on

- Dijon mustard

- 2 tbsp fresh lemon juice

Preparation

- Place walnuts in food processor; coarsely chop. Add breadcrumbs, lemon rind, olive oil and dill; pulse until crumbly. Mixture should stick together. Season with salt and pepper; set aside.

- Arrange salmon fillets skin side down on parchment paper lined baking sheets. Brush tops with mustard.

- Spoon 1/3 cup of walnut crumb mixture over each fillet; gently press the crumb mixture into the surface of the fish. Cover with plastic wrap; refrigerate for up to 2 hours.

- Bake at 350°F 15 to 20 minutes, or until salmon flakes with a fork. Just before serving, sprinkle each with 1 teaspoon lemon juice.

Mussels Three Ways

Mussels offer excellent nutrient density at a great value, making them an extremely accessible seafood. Avoid gritty mussels by soaking and rinsing them first, which allows tightly closed mussels to release any residual grit that the careless cook can miss. Because they're still alive, mussels are some of the freshest seafood in most stores.

Ingredients

With Heirloom Tomatoes and Pine Nut Topping

- 1 tablespoon olive oil

- 1/2 onion, minced

- 4 tomatoes, diced

- 2 pounds wild or farm-raised raw, tightly closed mussels

- 1 cup low-sodium chicken, vegetable, or beef broth

- 1/2 cup chopped fresh basil

- 1/2 cup pine nuts

With Garlicky Kale Ribbons and Artichokes

- 1 tablespoon olive oil

- 1/2 onion, minced

- 4 garlic cloves, thinly sliced

- 2 pounds wild or farm-raised raw, tightly closed mussels

- 4 large kale leaves, thinly sliced into ribbons

- 4 artichoke hearts, chopped

- 1 cup low-sodium chicken, vegetable, or beef broth

With White Wine and Roasted Red Pepper

- 1 tablespoon olive oil

- 1 onion, minced

- 2 pounds wild or farm-raised raw, tightly closed mussels

- 1/2 cup white wine

- 3/4 cup low-sodium chicken, vegetable, or beef broth

- 2 cups diced roasted red pepper

Directions

- Preparing mussels for cooking: Soak the mussels in a large bowl of cold water for 15 to 20 minutes. Using your fingers or a slotted spoon, lift out the mussels and transfer them to a colander. Rinse under cold running water several times and discard any mussels that are damaged or remain open after being firmly squeezed between your thumb and forefinger, or when you firmly tap them.

• Check each mussel for a threadlike string hanging out of the shell (called the "beard"). To remove, use a tea towel to grasp the beard, and pull firmly towards the hinge end of the shell and tug free.

Heirloom Tomatoes and Pine Nut Topping: Warm the olive oil in a large stockpot over medium heat. Add the onion and cook for 3 to 4 minutes until the onion begins to brown. Add the tomatoes and cook for 1 minute more until they begin to give off their liquid. Add the mussels and the broth. Cover and cook for 3 to 4 minutes until the mussels open and the meat inside is cooked through. Discard any mussels that have not opened. Sprinkle with the basil and pine nuts and serve immediately.

Garlicky Kale Ribbons and Artichokes: Warm the olive oil in a large stockpot over medium heat. Add the onion and garlic and cook for 3 to 4 minutes until the onion begins to brown. Add the mussels, kale, artichokes, and broth. Cover and cook 3 to 4 minutes until the mussels open and the meat inside is cooked through. Discard any mussels that have not opened. Serve immediately.

White Wine and Roasted Red Pepper: Warm the olive oil in a large stockpot over medium heat. Add the onion and cook for 3 to 4 minutes until the onion begins to brown. Add the mussels, wine, and broth. Cover and cook for 3 to 4 minutes until the muscles open and the meat inside is cooked through. Discard any mussels that have not opened. Sprinkle with the roasted red pepper and serve immediately.

Roasted Ginger Salmon

All I can say is get out your camera, cause when you make this dish, you're going to want to take a picture of it before you serve it. It's just that pretty, with the peach of the salmon, the ruby red jewels of the pomegranate seeds, the vibrant green of the parsley. The taste is no less sensational, the citrus and herbs playing wonderfully off the salmon's healthy blend of omega-3 rich fats. This one will energize all your senses.

Ingredients

- 1/2 cup freshly squeezed orange juice

- 2 tablespoons freshly squeezed lime juice

- 2 tablespoons freshly squeezed lemon juice

- Zest of 1 orange

- Zest of 1 lemon

- 1 tablespoon extra-virgin olive oil

- 1/2 teaspoon finely minced fresh ginger

- Pinch of cayenne pepper

- 4 (6-ounce) salmon fillets, pin bones removed

- Sea salt

- 1 teaspoon Dijon mustard

- 1 cup Pomegranate Olive Mint Salsa

Directions

- In a small bowl or glass measuring cup, whisk together the orange juice, lime juice, lemon juice, orange zest, lemon zest, olive oil, ginger, and cayenne. Place the salmon in a baking dish and season each piece with a pinch of salt.

Pour half of the marinade over the salmon and turn to coat well. Cover the baking dish and marinate in the refrigerator for 20 minutes.

• Preheat the oven to 400°F.

• Remove the salmon from the refrigerator, uncover, and add 2 tablespoons of water to the dish. Bake for 10 to 15 minutes, depending on the thickness of the fillets, just until tender and opaque and an instant-read thermometer inserted into the center of the fillet registers 120°F.

• While the salmon is cooking, combine the reserved marinade and the mustard in a small saucepan over medium heat and simmer until the liquid is reduced by half. Pour the reduction over the fillets. Spoon 1/4 cup of the relish on top of each fillet, and serve immediately.

COOK'S NOTE: Like Goldilocks and the three bears, fish has to be just right. Too much time in the oven or on the grill leaves your fish too dry. Too little time and you will have raw fish. As with many other proteins, fish continues to cook for several minutes after you take it off the heat. This is called carryover cooking. Let an instant read thermometer be your guide and pull your fish away from the heat at 120°F. By the time you're ready to serve it, your fish will be perfect.

Spinach And Cranberry Stuffed Salmon

Ingredients

- 1 lb. of Salmon fillets

- ½ cup of fresh spinach leaves

- 3 – 4 fresh basil leaves chopped

- 1 tsp lemon zest

- 1 clove of garlic minced

- 2 T craisins chopped

- 2 T nuts chopped (pecans, walnuts or almonds are recommended)

- 1 tsp of dried oregano

- 1 T Dijon Mustard

- ½ cup breadcrumbs

Directions

- Sauté the spinach, lemon zest, and garlic until spinach is wilted.

• Combine the craisins, nuts, basil, and oregano leaves in a small bowl. Add the wilted spinach mixture to the small bowl and combine.

• Cut a pocket horizontally into each salmon fillet. Stuff each pocket with about 2 tablespoons of the combined mixture.

• Spread 1 tablespoon of Dijon mustard on the salmon and finish by sprinkling breadcrumbs on top of each fillet.

• Place salmon on non-stick baking sheet or backing sheet lined with oven safe paper and bake for 20 minutes at 375° F or until fillets are fully cooked.

Triple-Citrus Ginger Black Cod

Shopping for fish can be intimidating.Maybe it's the fact that half of them are staring at you from behind the counter, as if to say, "Jeez, how did I end up here?" So, if you're going to do them—and yourself—justice, here's how to rustle up a fine, fresh fillet.You need to use your eyes and your nose. Look for a cut where the flesh is moist and glistening, with no flat, brown edges. If the fish looks dull, take a pass.Same goes for any fillet with a fishy or ammonia smell. Don't be shy about asking your fishmonger a few questions, like when the fish came in and from where. Most stores have regular shipments; knowing that schedule in advance can help you plan when to have fish. If black cod were in a band, it would be the bass player: steady, meaty, but not much of a soloist. It benefits from some jazzy front men and especially likes to swing with citrus high notes. You'll find plenty of those riffs in this dish.

Ingredients

- 1/2 cup freshly squeezed orange juice

- 2 tablespoons freshly squeezed lime juice

- 2 tablespoons freshly squeezed lemon juice

- 1 tablespoon extra-virgin olive oil

- Zest of 1 orange

- Zest of 1 lemon

- 1/2 teaspoon minced fresh ginger

- Pinch of cayenne

- 4 3.5-ounce black cod fillets, pin bones removed

- 1/2 teaspoon sea salt

- 1 teaspoon Dijon mustard

- 1/4 cup coarsely chopped fresh flat-leaf parsley or mint

COOK'S NOTE: This versatile, delicious marinade is great with other fish, such as sea bass, salmon, and halibut. These flavors also pair nicely with Warm Napa Cabbage Slaw. You can also cook the fish on a grill. Wipe the marinade off the fillets and rub them with 1 teaspoon of light sesame oil. Grill over low, even heat for about 4 minutes per side, until the flesh is opaque and flakes easily and the center of each fillet registers 137°F.

Directions

- In a small bowl or glass measuring cup, whisk together the orange juice, lime juice, lemon juice, olive oil, orange zest, lemon zest, ginger, and cayenne. Place the cod in a baking dish and season each piece with 1/8 teaspoon of the salt. Pour half of the orange juice mixture over the cod and turn to coat well. Cover and marinate in the refrigerator for 30 minutes.

- Preheat the oven to 400°F.

• Remove the cod from the refrigerator, uncover, and add 2 tablespoons of water to the bottom of the dish. Bake just until the fillets are tender and an instant-read thermometer inserted into the center of each fillet registers 137°F; it will take 10 to 15 minutes, depending on the thickness of the fillets.

• Meanwhile, combine the remaining orange juice mixture and the mustard in a small saucepan over medium heat and simmer until the liquid is reduced by half. Pour the reduction over the fillets, sprinkle with the parsley, and serve immediately.

STORAGE: Store tightly wrapped in an airtight container in the refrigerator for 1 to 2 days.

Arugula, Strawberry And Walnut Salad
Ingredients

Salad

• 2 cups arugula

• 1 red endive, thinly sliced (1/4-inch rings)

• 1/2 cup California walnuts, candied

• 2 ounces walnut oil

- 2 ounces Pickled Shallots

- 8 strawberries, sliced

Candied Walnuts

- 1/2 cup California walnuts

- 1 egg white

- 1-ounce sugar or sugar substitute

- 2 tablespoons walnut oil

- Salt to taste

Pickled Shallots

- 2 shallots, medium, sliced

- 4 ounces red wine vinegar

- 1-ounce sugar or sugar substitute

- Salt to taste

Preparation

- For the candied walnuts, beat egg white until it forms soft peaks. Add the sugar or sugar substitute and mix together. Add the walnuts and coat with the egg mixture. Place in a

300°F oven for 30 minutes, stirring every 10 minutes. Allow to cool. Once mixture is cool, toss in walnut oil.

• For the pickled shallots, bring vinegar, sugar or sugar substitute and salt up to a simmer in a saucepan and pour over sliced shallots. Allow to cool.

• To make the salad combine all ingredients, using the vinegar from the shallots and walnut oil from the walnuts as the vinaigrette. Serve immediately.

Barley Stuffed Tomato With Caramelized Vegetables

Barley is an under-appreciated cereal grain with a pasta-like consistency and high fiber content. With its fiber it aids in optimizing the good bacteria in the intestines reducing the risk of colon cancer and hemorrhoids. Topped with light pecorino cheese and a placed in a colorful tomato "bowl", this recipe will soon become a summer favorite.

Ingredients

• 1 cup barley

• 2 1/2 cups vegetable stock

• 1 tbsp olive oil

• 6 oz artichoke hearts, sliced thin

- 1 small red onion, sliced

- 1 small bulb fennel, sliced thin

- 4 cloves garlic, minced

- 1 tbsp dry red pepper flakes

- 1/4 cup white wine

- 1/4 cup pecorino cheese, shredded

- 1/4 cup assorted minced herbs

- 3 large tomatoes, cut in 1/2 from top to bottom, seeds removed to form vessel

Directions

- In a dry pot over low heat, toast barley until golden. Add vegetable stock and cook until barley is al dente, about 20 to 30 minutes. Set aside.

- In a large sauté pan, add olive oil and warm over high heat until oil is almost smoking. Carefully add artichoke hearts, red onion, and fennel. Sauté, stirring constantly until caramelization begins to occur.

• Add garlic and red pepper flakes and continue cooking until fragrant. Deglaze pant with white wine.

• Remove from heat, add to cooked barley, and stir in pecorino and herbs. Season to taste and set aside to cool to room temperature.

• Stuff halved tomatoes with the barley and vegetable mixture and serve at room temperature with a drizzle of olive oil and a sprinkle of minced herbs.

Brandon's Roasted Broccoli

They say kids don't like vegetables, but my grandson Brandon evidently didn't get that memo. He's eaten and loved veggies since the age of two (he's eight now), with broccoli being his favorite. He's not shy about it, either. Last time he was over I asked him how he wanted his broccoli. He said, "Roasted... where you lay them out on a cookie sheet." Want a scene that'll melt your heart? That's watching Brandon down on all fours, peering through the glass into the oven at his broccoli baking. When they come out, I put a little Parmesan cheese on top, and Brandon's picking them off the roasting pan.

Ingredients

- 2 1/2 pounds broccoli, cut into florets with 2 inches of trimmed stem

- 2 tablespoons extra-virgin olive oil

- 1 tablespoon minced garlic

- 1/2 teaspoon sea salt

- 1/4 teaspoon freshly ground black pepper

- 1 teaspoon lemon zest

- 1/4 cup Parmesan cheese (optional)

- 1 tablespoon chopped fresh basil (optional)

- Freshly squeezed lemon juice

Directions

- Position a rack in the middle of the oven and preheat the oven to 400°F. Line a rimmed baking sheet with parchment paper.

- Put the broccoli, olive oil, garlic, salt, pepper, and lemon zest in a large bowl and toss until the broccoli is evenly coated. Transfer to the lined baking sheet and spread it in an even layer. Bake for 15 to 20 minutes, until the broccoli begins to brown and is tender.

• Transfer to a bowl, add the lemon zest, Parmesan, and basil, and toss to combine. Add a spritz of lemon juice and serve immediately.

COOK'S NOTE: Be sure to add the lemon juice and zest just before serving, as the lemon will dull the color of the broccoli if it sits for more than just a few minutes.

Latin Style Kale

With Latin American greens, it's all in the seeds. In this case, toasted cumin and pumpkin seeds (a.k.a. pepitas) along with a hit of lime juice give this kale a breezy, fresh Latin feel.

Ingredients

• 8 cups, stemmed and chopped dino kale in bite size pieces

• 2 tablespoons extra virgin olive oil

• 2 1/2 cups or one medium red onion, cut into half moons

• Sea salt

• 3 cloves garlic, minced

- 1/4 teaspoon cumin seeds, (toasted)

- Pinch of cayenne

- 1 teaspoon lemon zest

- 1 1/2 teaspoon freshly squeezed lemon juice

- 1 1/2 teaspoon freshly squeezed lime juice

- 1/2 teaspoon Grade A Dark Amber organic maple syrup

- 2 tablespoon toasted pepitas (garnish)

Directions

- Cover the kale with cold water and set aside.

- Heat the olive oil in a large, deep sauté pan over medium-high heat, then add the onion, a pinch of salt and sauté for 3 minutes. Decrease the heat to low and cook slowly until the onions are caramelized.

- While the onions are caramelizing toast the cumin seeds in a small pan over medium heat, shaking a few times for even toasting until they become aromatic and start to brown slightly. Transfer to a small bowl and set aside. In the same pan, add the peptias, shaking the pan for even toasting, until they become aromatic. Transfer to a small bowl and reserve.

• Increase the heat to medium; add the garlic, cumin, pinch of cayenne and pinch of salt and sauté for 3 to 4 minutes. Drain the kale and add it to the pan. Sauté until the greens turn bright green and wilt, about 4 minutes. While the greens are cooking whisk together the lemon, orange juice, zests and maple syrup together. Test the greens and continue cooking, covered until they become a little more tender. Drizzle with the citrus maple mixture. Top with the toasted pepitas.

Sweet And Sour Sesame Asian Cabbage And Kale

Here's a classic sweet-and-sour taste with a mouth-watering, eye-catching twist. Tamari, ginger, and toasted sesame oil combine with lime juice to bring the Great Wall to your great room. And cabbage? That's another super food that's a must-have on the plate.

Ingredients

• 1 teaspoon freshly grated ginger

• 1 tablespoon plus 2 teaspoons tamari (wheat free soy sauce)

- 1 tablespoon lime juice

- 1 tablespoon Grade A Dark Amber maple syrup

- 1 teaspoon toasted sesame oil

- 2 tablespoons extra virgin olive oil

- 4 cups kale, washed, stems removed and cut into bite size pieces

- Sea Salt

- 2 cups red cabbage, shredded

- 1 tablespoon sesame seeds toasted

Directions

- In a small bowl combine the ginger, tamari, lime juice, maple syrup and toasted sesame oil and set aside.

- Place a small skillet over a low flame and toast the sesame seeds until they turn slightly brown and smell nutty, about 1 minute. Remove to a plate.

- Heat the olive oil in a large, deep sauté pan over medium –high heat, then add the kale, and a pinch of salt and sauté for 2 minutes. Add the cabbage, and another pinch of salt, sauté for 1 more minute. Add the sauce and cook for 2 more minutes or until tender. Add the toasted sesame seeds. Serve immediately.

Indian Greens

This meal in bowl is filled with fiber and protein from chickpeas and packs flavor that simply has to be experienced to be believed. Coconut milk, curry, turmeric…it's all a taste bud blast with outrageous anti-inflammatory ingredients.

Ingredients

• 2 tablespoons extra virgin olive oil

• 1/4 teaspoon cumin seeds

• 1/4 teaspoon mustard seeds

• 1 teaspoon freshly grated ginger

• 1/2 teaspoon turmeric

• 1/8 teaspoon freshly ground black pepper

• 1/4 teaspoon curry powder

• 8 cups of Swiss chard, stems removed and torn into bite size pieces

- Sea Salt

- 1 cup garbanzo beans, drained and spritzed with lemon juice and a pinch of salt

- 1 cup organic diced canned tomatoes, reserve the juice

- 1/4 cup coconut milk

- 1/4 teaspoon Grade A Dark Amber maple syrup

Directions

- Cover the chard with cold water and set aside. Heat the olive oil in a large, deep sauté pan over medium –high heat, then add the mustard seeds and cumin seeds and sauté until they begin to pop, then add the ginger. Add the Swiss chard, a pinch of salt, turmeric, pepper, ginger, curry powder and 2 tablespoons of the reserved tomato juice and sauté for 2 minutes. Stir in the garbanzo beans and the tomatoes and sauté for 3 minutes more. Add the coconut milk and maple syrup. Serve immediately.

COOK'S NOTE: If you don't have cumin, mustard seeds or turmeric handy, sauté the chard with the ginger and add 2 teaspoons of curry powder.

Mediterranean Greens

This is like a taking a two-week cruise around the isles: we go Greek with olives and feta, Sicilian with—surprise—currants, and we'll give the Cypriots credit for the garlic and the mint. Plus, a double dose of citrus in the form of lemon and orange zest.

Ingredients

- 2 tablespoons extra virgin olive oil

- 2 cloves garlic, minced

- Pinch of red chili pepper flakes

- 6 cups, stemmed and chopped dino kale in bite size pieces

- Sea salt

- 1/4 cup kalamata olives, sliced

- 1 tablespoons currants

- 1 teaspoon orange zest

- 1 teaspoon freshly squeezed orange juice

- 2 teaspoons lemon zest

- 2 teaspoons freshly squeezed lemon juice

- 1/8 of a teaspoon freshly grated nutmeg

- 1/2 teaspoon Grade A Dark Amber organic maple syrup

- 1/4 cup goat or sheep's milk feta cheese

- 2 teaspoons freshly chopped mint (garnish)

Directions

- Cover the kale with cold water and set aside. In a small bowl whisk together the lemon and orange juice, zests, nutmeg and maple syrup, then add the currents and allow them to soak. Reserve.

- Heat the olive oil in a large, deep sauté pan over medium heat, add the garlic and chili pepper flakes, sauté until the garlic turns lightly golden, about 20 seconds. Drain the kale and add it to the pan along with a scant quarter teaspoon of salt and 1 tablespoon of water. Sauté until the greens turn bright green and wilt, about 4 minutes. Add the soaked currents, along with their soaking liquid and the olives, and sauté until the greens become a little more tender. Turn off the heat, sprinkle in the feta cheese and garnish with the mint. Serve immediately.

Golden Roasted Cauliflower

My dad was in the salad dressing business, and that meant we never knew what kind of science experiment might show up on the dinner table. One day it might be a new Roquefort dressing, the next day a zesty ranch concoction. There were always plenty of raw veggies available for dipping, and dad's favorite was raw cauliflower with Thousand Island dressing. In fact, for years I just assumed the only way anyone ate cauliflower was raw.

I'm glad I know better now. Roasting cauliflower completely transforms it into a candy-like delight that yields to a gentle fork. The spices in this recipe—cumin, coriander, and turmeric—really make it sing. All have health benefits, but turmeric is a superstar: it has anticancer and anti-inflammatory properties and holds great promise for maintaining, and possibly even improving, brain health.

Ingredients

- 1 medium head of cauliflower (about 2 1/2 to 3 pounds) cut into 1 1/2-inch florets (about 8 cups)

- 2 tablespoons of extra virgin olive oil

- 1/2 teaspoon sea salt

- 1/4 teaspoon freshly ground pepper

- 1/2 teaspoon cumin

- 1/4 teaspoon coriander

- 1/2 teaspoon turmeric

- 1 tablespoon minced garlic

- 1 teaspoon lemon juice

- 1 tablespoon finely chopped parsley or cilantro

Directions

- Place the rack in the middle of the oven and preheat to 450°F. Line a baking sheet with parchment paper.

- Toss the cauliflower with 2 tablespoons olive oil, salt, pepper, cumin, coriander, turmeric and garlic. Spread the cauliflower mixture in an even layer on the prepared pan. Bake until the cauliflower is golden and tender, about 25 to 35 minutes. Toss with spritz with fresh lemon juice and parsley or cilantro.

Ikarian Tabouli Salad

Ikaria's traditional diet, like that found in much of the Mediterranean, includes a lot of vegetables and olive oil, small amounts of dairy and meat products, and moderate amounts of alcohol. Its emphasis on legumes, wild greens and olive oil contribute to the island's extreme longevity. Tabouli is a traditional Mediterranean dish that features parsley as the star of the show. The secret to a traditional Ikarian tabouli is the ratio of bulgar to parsley. Be sure you have a tabouli salad with a little bit of bulgar, not a bowl of bulgar with a little bit of salad.

Ingredients

- 1/3 cup bulgur wheat, rinsed

- 5 bunches parsley, finely chopped

- 5 medium tomatoes, diced small

- 1/2 cup chopped green onions

- 3 lemons, freshly squeezed

- 1/4 cup mint

- 1/2 cup extra-virgin olive oil

- 1/2 tbsp salt, or to taste

- 1/2 tsp pepper, or to taste

Directions

• Mix all ingredients together and enjoy.

Note: This also makes a great leftover salad.

Made in the USA
Las Vegas, NV
06 December 2023